* ARTHRITIS *

• •

NATUROPATHIC ADVICE TO HELP and PREVENT.

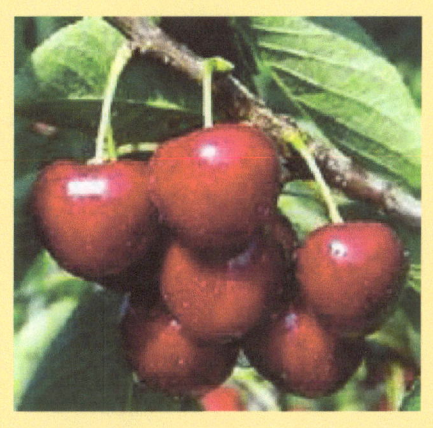

Written by: SHEILA BER – Naturopathic Consultant.

INTRODUCTION:

I'm a Microbiological/Chemical Technologist, who is currently working as a Naturopathic Consultant.

I'm writing this book to provide advice and help, to treat and prevent Arthritis and related problems, by removing the root causes, rather than addressing the symptom only.

There are many internal and external factors, influencing the body and affecting how you feel, think, act, eat. These are all manifested often times also into arthritic pain that causes unnecessary suffering.

Much of the advice provided in this book, is from my micro-biological/chemical background, as well as from my own personal experience.

I dedicate the book to both my sons: Bernard and Philip. Particularly also to all who seek simple, natural and effective treatment to eliminate any Arthritic symptoms and the pain associated with it.

INDEX:

There are many types of arthritis, ranging from osteoarthritis to rheumatoid arthritis. Osteoarthritis is characterized by the wear and tear of cartilage. Rheumatoid arthritis, on the other hand, is the inflammation of the joints resulting from a viral infection or autoimmune response.

Although the actual cause of arthritis is still not completely known, several potential causes can be due to: injuries, infections, abnormal metabolism, and/or an overactive immune system.

Due to the various causes, treatment programs would therefore focus on the specific causes. Arthritis common symptoms are: pain, fever, joint stiffness, warmth, redness, and swelling. Moreover, deformities may result from the limited joint functions. If left untreated, other organs of the body such as the kidneys, heart, and lungs may get affected.

MY BEST ADVICE TO YOU:

The basic causes contributing to Arthritis are as following:

1) High microbial activity that results in inflammation.

Take Probiotics! They have many health benefits, and they help fight and eliminate the microbes, that cause inflammation.

Daily elimination of chemical and microbial toxins. Toxins circulate in your body, impacting your joints negatively, causing inflammation, pain, and swelling. Daily elimination help reduce all of these symptoms.

2) *<u>Mechanical action</u>* of the joints, and cartilage erosion.
Cartilage acts as insulation between the bones. Causes vary, and include wear and tear: constant use, overuse or wrong use of the joints, that increase the risk of damage to them.

Minimize wearing high heels. Wear comfortable shoes that provide you with an adequate support.
Check also your body balance. Imbalanced body affects the way you walk, and thus affects also the mechanical function of your knees. If you feel that you are lacking balance, see a Chiropractor, or a Physiotherapist. You may need to adjust your back and posture periodically.

*Exercise: Doing daily exercises, within your comfortable limits, with a little challenge or resistance, will help you build endurance, balance, and mobility.

Please see clause
#10 below, for further information.

3) <u>Pressure</u> - Exerting pressure from heavy weight, on joints, particularly the knees, can contribute to further damage and erosion of the cartilage, tendons and the bones .Do not carry heavy weights. Handle weight that you feel is light, and that will not exert pressure on your knees.
Your knees carry big part of your body weight.

If you are overweight, you will benefit greatly from losing weight that feels comfortable to you, and that also will benefit your knees, and other joints.

4) <u>Temperature</u> - Keep your joints warm, especially the knees during cool and cold seasons.

The knees are very sensitive to cold. Cold temperature aggravates and stiffens them, as well as all other joints, resulting in inflammation and pain, particularly if you are already suffering from some degree of Arthritis. <u>Solution</u>: Wear leg warmers, that can be pulled over your knees, day and night, to ensure that they are kept constantly warm!

*You can obtain Acrylic leg warmers at most Dollarama stores, at a very low price.

Note: Keeping the knees warm, when the temperature of your surrounding is under 15 °C, makes a world of a difference, to how your knees feel!

5) <u>Moisture</u> - High humidity level in the air, and lower barometric pressure represent unfavourable environment for Arthritic sufferers.

*Take care of your joints, especially the knees, by applying a barrier on the area of the joints.

<u>Solution</u>: A suitable barrier can be any ordinary, healthy cooking oil, such as Grape Seed, Almond, Mustard, or even Canola oil. Massage daily, any of the above on the joint area, for a few seconds. The oil will leave a layer, that will keep moisture out.

Additionally, oils that are rich in Anti-Oxidants, when penetrating the skin, will provide your joints with excellent health benefits, as well as with much needed lubrication.

6) **Imbalanced body pH**. **Your blood pH has to be slightly alkaline**, and if it is acidic, it gives rise to higher microbial activity in your body, oxygen deprivation, thus higher inflammation level, that manifests itself in many ways.

Overall body pH has a significant effect on all joints, organs, blood vessels, tissues, hormones, in short, all body systems. Acidic pH is attributed to **high** consumption of sugars/carbohydrates, proteins, oils and fats, and stress.

To alkalize daily do the following: Take 1/2 tsp Baking Soda (Arm & Hammer) in 1 cup water, with 1 Potassium tablet. You may need to repeat the above 2-3 times a day, so that your body will be slightly alkaline: pH 7.0-7.5.

To test your body pH, you simply test the pH in your urine, as following:
A simple test is done with a Q-Tip (coated with Turmeric, and has light yellow color) and is placed under the stream of urine.
If the pH is acidic, it will remain yellow, and if it is alkaline, the color of the Q-Tip will appear in color ranging from orange to red wine color.

Orange to red wine, are the colors that you have to obtain. If you see yellow on your Q-tip, immediately, alkalize, by taking your Baking Soda drink, as described above.

**To prepare your Q-Tips for the test, do the following simple steps: In a small container, place several tablespoons of rubbing Ethyl alcohol (S.D.M Pharmacy.). Mix in: 1/2 teaspoon Turmeric powder. Mix well. Immerse 10-20 Q-Tips in the mixture.

Let dry over a piece of paper. Cut them in 1/2, so you can use both ends for more tests. You'll have a month supply to do your daily pH tests.

7) <u>Electrolyte imbalance</u>- If your body electrolyte fluids are not balanced, the electrical conductivity in your joints is not optimal. Thus resulting in less of the following:

blood circulation, oxygen , nutrients and energy.

To balance your electrolytes take daily: Multi-minerals, and also 1 Potassium tablet 99 mg - 1-2x a day.

8) <u>Diet</u> - Diet that consists of excessive sugars, carbohydrates and junk foods that contain also unhealthy oils and fats, that may be harmful and toxic to your joints, and body in general.

Diets high sugars in any form, including carbohydrates (carbs), will feed the anaerobic bacteria and yeast in your body, multiplying them and increasing the microbial level, that will result in inflammation and pain, consequently erosion of joints cartilage, and bones.

Reduce your sugars/carbs intake!

*Note: Honey (monosaccharides) in moderation is good.
It breaks down and gets absorbed more rapidly, allowing less time for microbes to feed and multiply.

Honey can be used in coffee, tea, baking, and more.
It is kept at room temperature, but has to be handled carefully, by always using clean utensils during usage, to prevent any microbial contamination.

9) <u>Mental state</u> - If you are experiencing stress that is extreme, or if your emotions are fluctuating, out of control. It is individual, and each person extreme varies, according to their coping capabilities.

Find positive ways to deal with it, and do not let it linger, as it is harmful to your health, and your joints will feel it!

Stress converts body pH to acidic as following:

HIGHER STRESS LEVEL = INCREASED BODY ACIDITY.

INCREASED ACIDITY = HIGHER MICROBIAL LEVEL.

HIGHER MICROBIAL LEVEL = INCREASED INFLAMMATION AND PAIN!

GREATER RELAXATION = DECREASED BODY ACIDITY.

DECREASED ACIDITY = DECREASED INFLAMMATION AND PAIN!

ALKALIZE DAILY!   See clause #6 above.

When body pH is very acidic, it impedes normal metabolic activities, resulting in inflammation and pain.

*Body acidity is detected in blood and urine, as well as in saliva.

TO ARREST THE PROGRESSION OF ARTHRITIS IN YOUR JOINTS, take the following daily:

1) GLS-500 - (Glucosamine Sulfate)or GLS-1000, 1 capsule - 2x a day.

You may take GLS with food, if experiencing any discomfort.

*Give it time to have full effect: 3-4 weeks!

2) **Boswellia** - An anti-inflammatory herb that is very effective. 1 tablet 2x a day.

3) **MSM** - (Methylsulfonylmethane) 1000 mg. - excellent in reducing pain and inflammation. Take 1 capsule 2x a day. For increased pain and inflammation, you may safely take 1-6 capsules 3x a day, preferably on empty stomach.

4) **Multi-vitamins.**

5) **B-Complex** - 1 tablet - 1-2x daily, with food, to help with stress.

6) *Vitamin D3* - 4,000- 6,000 I.U. caplets, 2x daily, taken with Omega oil/Flax oil for maximum absorption. Vitamin D is a steroid anti-inflammatory.

It is very beneficial particularly in higher concentration, for keeping inflammation down.

It maintains healthy bones, and balanced Thyroid. Vitamin D3 can be safely taken, up to 10,000 I.U. a day. Improvement in health, and reduction in inflammation, is noticed immediately.

7) *Beta Carotene* - 1 caplet 2x a day, with food. It helps to fight inflammation!!!
It converts to vitamin A, and is stored in the liver.

8) <u>Cod liver oil</u> – *Cod liver oil is highly anti inflammatory, as it high in the following: vitamin A & D, omega 3, EPA and DHA. The oil has many health benefits. I cannot emphasize enough, how helpful it is in reducing inflammation and pain in the joints, as well as throughout the body. Take 2-4 tablespoon liquid oil a day, before or after meals. Cod liver oil also reduces body cholesterol level, helps with clearing inflammation from the lungs, and it alleviates symptoms of depression!*

9) *Aspirin - 81 mg <u>coated</u> - even every other day. Take it with food only! It is very effective in reducing inflammation.*

You can verify this by checking your blood ESR (Erythrocyte sedimentation rate) level, when taking a blood test.

10) Calcium Citrate - This form is more absorbable. Take 1,200 -1,500 mg a day, along with vitamin C, to further aid absorption, to maintain strong bones.

11) Enzymes – They promote better metabolism, And aid in digestion. Enzyme treatments for curing Arthritis have by far produced more positive results.
The use of <u>proteolytic enzymes</u> such as Serrapeptase has shown that these enzymes are capable of dissolving dead or scar tissues without harming the healthy living tissues.

They are much safer alternative for steroidal and non steroidal inflammatory drugs such as NSAIDs. They are also considered <u>a safer option</u> over any exotic treatment.

12) Coenzyme Q10 – Coenzymes are essential organic compounds that attach to enzymes to help them catalyze all reactions. Coenzyme Q10 boost the immune system, and helps with the production of energy.

13) Cherries – the berries are very helpful in lowering inflammation, and they are rich in many vitamins including A,C, and Potassium. They assist in reducing body acidity. You can have them fresh or in any other form. Cherry syrup diluted in a 1 glass of water, is also helpful.

14) Copper bracelet- Copper is believed to have antioxidant properties to prevent free radicals from damaging joints. Copper is gradually absorbed through the skin, relieving pain. You can wear it day and night. It works!

15) Exercise & Yoga - You must exercise daily, 15-20 minutes, to keep your joints, as well as your muscles from getting stiff. If you don't, you will experience poor mobility.

When you mobilize or work your joints and muscles, your body secrets essential biochemical lubricating fluids, gradually helping you to reach optimum mobility.

<u>NOTE</u>: Even if you are experiencing great pain, make your best efforts to exercise. You will only feel better later, as the pain eventually subsides!

Lubricating fluids slowly make it easier to exercise. If you are in extreme pain, you may take Tylenol, 1/2 hour before the workout.

Yoga - Doing yoga even 10-15 minutes a day, lying on your back comfortably, will provide you with many health benefits, physically, mentally, and spiritually.

You can check some of the exercises in the following websites:

http://www.ehow.com/way_5344176_top-yoga-exercises-hip-pain.html

and

http://www.livestrong.com/article/419696-gentle-exercises-when-lying-down/

I hope you find the above information very helpful.

BER SHEILA, 2012.

Disclaimer

SHEILA BER BIOGRAPHY   2012.

Professionally:

I'm a **Microbiological/Chemical Technologist**, currently working as a **Naturopathic consultant**.
I worked in Microbiology and Chemistry, for about 12 years, in the Pharmaceutical, cosmetics, and toiletry industries.

I started out as a microbiological/Chemical Analyst. I Performed:
chemical and microbiological analysis of raw materials, finished products, variety of packaging materials and their compatibility with different range of finished products.

Chemical analysis tests were carried out with up to date technologically advanced instruments, such as Spectrophotometers, and other apparatus. Microbiological tests including incubation of samples, and microscopical studies of a variety of bacteria, yeast, and fungus.

I was also involved in Research & Development, and in formulations of large variety of products. I've carried out many formulations, and modified some when required.

I've advanced several years later, to a higher position with the title of Quality Control Manager.

My work included:

1) Quality Control of raw materials, finished products, packaging.

2) I was responsible for managing and supporting the laboratory personnel.

3) Additionally, I have carried out inspections on the production floor facilities, the equipment, including ventilation system, and other systems. Monthly reporting on the findings, my recommendations, and implementation of required corrective actions.

4) Communication with Health Canada, particularly to obtain their regulatory approvals for new patents and new products. Providing them with documentation, and MSDS information of the raw material involved, in all the formulations.
I have tremendously enjoyed all the above duties.

It's very technically involved work, very interesting, and challenging.

Personally:

Generally, I'm rather unconventional, though as getting older, I become slightly more conventional. I like things straight simple, uncomplicated!
I like helping people. I try to view things, situations, from different perspectives.

I refrain from judging others, but need to know all the facts and reasons for their particular behaviour, thoughts and actions, before forming any opinion.
I take everything with a grain of salt, always stay alert, and cautious.

Life has its highs and lows, but I always try to stay afloat. Trying is the key word!

I often check my expectations, and may lower them at times, to keep things in perspective.

At the age of 20, I've completed 2 years of service, in the ARMY, filling the position of Sergeant. It was definitely, a significant lifetime experience for me.

I have two grown up sons. I love them very dearly! I enjoy being a caring mother, not perfect, with always room for improvement.

EDUCATION:

*I've graduated with **Honours in Science,** and with **Distinction in Physics.***

Seneca College
Microbiological/Chemical Technology

Technical school
Architecture/Mechanical Drafting

School of Accounting
General Accounting

OCCUPATION:

I'm currently working as a Naturopathic Consultant.

EMPLOYMENT HISTORY:

DRUG TRADING COMPANY - Toronto
Microbiological/Chemical Technologist

FABERGE - Toronto
Quality Control/ Laboratory Manager

REVLON - Toronto
Quality Control/ Laboratory Manager

ACCENTURE Business for Utilities - Toronto
Accounting/Administration

I *Lived in:*
1) Toronto, Canada,

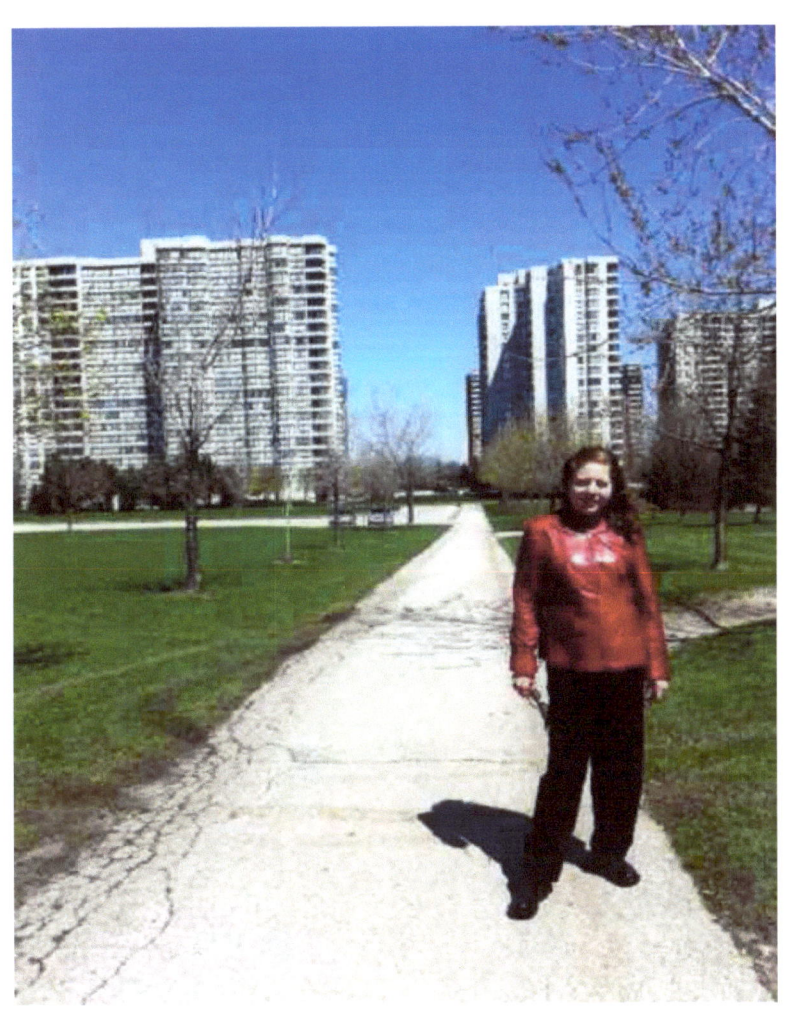

SHEILA BER, 2012.

(SHULLA)

Disclaimer.

ALKALIZE and SURVIVE!

www.ingramcontent.com/pod-product-compliance
Lightning Source LLC
Chambersburg PA
CBHW050911290526
45792CB00002B/769